THE COMPLETE 2024 HYPOTHYROIDISM DIET COOKBOOK

100+ Nutritional Recipes for Healing of Hypothyroidism and Hashimoto's with Delicious Meal Plan to Lose Weight and Boost Energy

LUCKY WILSON

CONTENTS

INTRODUCTION

Understanding Hypothyroidism

Hypothyroidism, often referred to as an underactive thyroid, is a condition where the thyroid gland fails to produce sufficient amounts of thyroid hormones. These hormones, including thyroxine (T4) and triiodothyronine (T3), play a crucial role in regulating metabolism, energy production, and overall bodily functions. When these hormones are deficient, various physiological processes slow down, leading to symptoms such as fatigue, weight gain, cold intolerance, depression, and cognitive impairments.

The thyroid gland, a small butterfly-shaped gland located at the base of the neck, is a vital component of the endocrine system. It receives signals from the pituitary gland, which releases thyroid-stimulating hormone (TSH) to prompt the production of T3 and T4. In hypothyroidism, this communication pathway is disrupted, often due to autoimmune conditions like Hashimoto's thyroiditis, where the immune system mistakenly attacks the thyroid tissue, leading to inflammation and reduced hormone production.

While genetic predisposition plays a role, other factors such as nutritional deficiencies, stress, certain medications, and exposure to environmental toxins can also contribute to the development of hypothyroidism. Diagnosing hypothyroidism typically involves blood tests to measure levels of TSH and thyroid hormones, along with an assessment of symptoms. Managing hypothyroidism often requires lifelong treatment with synthetic thyroid hormones, but dietary and lifestyle interventions can significantly enhance the quality of life and symptom management.

The Role of Diet in Managing Hypothyroidism

Diet plays a pivotal role in managing hypothyroidism and supporting thyroid health. Certain nutrients are essential for the synthesis and conversion of thyroid hormones. For instance, iodine is a critical component of T3 and T4, and selenium is necessary for the conversion of T4 to the more active T3 form. Deficiencies in these and other nutrients like zinc, vitamin D, and B vitamins can exacerbate hypothyroidism symptoms.

Conversely, certain foods can interfere with thyroid function. Goitrogens, found in cruciferous vegetables like broccoli and cauliflower, can inhibit iodine uptake when consumed in large quantities, particularly when raw. However, cooking these vegetables can reduce their goitrogenic effects. Additionally, gluten and soy products may affect thyroid function in susceptible individuals, and reducing or eliminating these from the diet can sometimes improve symptoms.

A well-balanced diet rich in whole foods, lean proteins, healthy fats, and a variety of fruits and vegetables can help manage hypothyroidism. Antioxidant-rich foods, such as berries and leafy greens, can combat oxidative stress, which is often elevated in individuals with thyroid disorders. Moreover, staying hydrated and maintaining regular eating patterns can support metabolic processes and energy levels.

Incorporating thyroid-supportive foods into your diet, such as seaweed for iodine, Brazil nuts for selenium, and fatty fish for omega-3 fatty acids, can make a significant difference. It's also important to avoid processed foods, excessive sugar, and trans fats, which can exacerbate inflammation and hinder thyroid function. By making mindful dietary choices, you can support your thyroid health and alleviate many of the symptoms associated with hypothyroidism.

Benefits of the Hypothyroidism Diet

1. Supports Thyroid Function: The diet focuses on nutrient-dense foods that support optimal thyroid function. It includes foods rich in iodine, selenium, and zinc, essential minerals for thyroid hormone production and regulation.

2. Manages Weight: Individuals with hypothyroidism often struggle with weight gain or difficulty losing weight. The diet emphasizes balanced meals that promote satiety and regulate metabolism, aiding in weight management goals.

3. Reduces Inflammation: Many foods in the hypothyroidism diet are anti-inflammatory, helping to

reduce inflammation levels in the body. Chronic inflammation is linked to various health issues and can exacerbate symptoms of thyroid disorders.

4. Improves Energy Levels: By providing balanced nutrition and stabilizing blood sugar levels, the diet helps combat fatigue and boosts energy throughout the day. This is crucial for individuals experiencing low energy due to thyroid dysfunction.

5. Enhances Nutrient Absorption: Certain nutrients, such as vitamins A, D, E, and K, are crucial for thyroid health and are better absorbed when consumed with a balanced diet rich in healthy fats, lean proteins, and fiber.

6. Supports Digestive Health: The diet promotes gut health through the inclusion of probiotic-rich foods like yogurt and kefir, as well as fiber from fruits, vegetables, and whole grains. A healthy gut contributes to overall well-being and can aid in nutrient absorption.

7. Regulates Hormones: Hormonal balance is crucial for thyroid health. The diet emphasizes foods that support hormone regulation and metabolism, helping to stabilize hormone levels and reduce symptoms associated with hormonal imbalances.

8. Promotes Heart Health: Many aspects of the hypothyroidism diet, such as reducing processed foods and incorporating heart-healthy fats like omega-3s from fish and nuts, contribute to cardiovascular health. This is important as individuals with hypothyroidism may be at higher risk for heart disease.

9. Supports Mental Well-being: Proper nutrition plays a vital role in mental health. The diet includes foods rich in vitamins and minerals that support cognitive function and mood stability, helping to alleviate symptoms of depression and brain fog often associated with thyroid disorders.

10. Customizable and Sustainable: The hypothyroidism diet can be tailored to individual preferences and dietary restrictions, making it adaptable and sustainable for long-term health management.

How to Use This Cookbook for Optimal Thyroid Health

This cookbook is designed to be your comprehensive guide to managing hypothyroidism through nutritious and delicious meals. It aims to simplify the often overwhelming process of dietary adjustments by providing you with a collection of recipes that are not only thyroid-friendly but also satisfying and enjoyable. Here's how to make the most out of this cookbook:

1. Understand the Nutritional Basis: Each recipe in this cookbook has been crafted with a keen understanding of the nutritional needs specific to hypothyroidism. We've focused on incorporating ingredients that support thyroid function, such as iodine-rich sea vegetables, selenium-packed nuts and seeds, and anti-inflammatory herbs and spices. The recipes are designed to provide a balance of macronutrients—proteins, fats, and carbohydrates—while emphasizing micronutrients vital for thyroid health.

2. Follow the Meal Plans: To make your journey smoother, we've included meal plans tailored to different needs, whether you're looking to lose weight, boost your energy

levels, or simply maintain a healthy thyroid. These meal plans offer a structured approach, ensuring that you get a variety of nutrients throughout the week without the stress of planning every meal from scratch.

3. Adapt to Your Lifestyle: We understand that everyone's lifestyle and preferences are unique. Therefore, the recipes are flexible and adaptable. Feel free to adjust portion sizes, swap ingredients, and make modifications to suit your dietary needs and taste preferences. We've also included tips on how to make quick substitutions without compromising the nutritional value of the meals.

4. Mindful Cooking Techniques: The way you prepare your food can impact its nutritional value. We've included cooking techniques that preserve nutrient integrity, such as steaming, sautéing, and baking, while minimizing methods that can degrade essential nutrients. Additionally, we've highlighted the importance of using quality ingredients, such as organic produce and grass-fed meats, to reduce exposure to toxins that can interfere with thyroid function.

5. Monitor Your Progress: Keeping track of how you feel after incorporating these recipes into your diet is crucial. Pay attention to changes in your energy levels, mood,

weight, and other symptoms. This can help you identify which foods and recipes work best for you. We've included spaces for notes and reflections to help you monitor your progress and make necessary adjustments.

6. Stay Informed and Inspired: Managing hypothyroidism is a lifelong journey, and staying informed about the latest research and nutritional insights can empower you to make the best choices for your health. This cookbook is more than just a collection of recipes; it's a resource that offers guidance, inspiration, and support. Explore the additional tips, reading materials, and resources provided to deepen your understanding of hypothyroidism and its management.

By using this cookbook, you are taking a proactive step towards better thyroid health. Remember, the goal is not just to manage hypothyroidism but to thrive and enjoy a vibrant, energetic life. With the right nutritional strategies and delicious recipes at your disposal, you can achieve optimal thyroid health and overall well-being.

The Fundamentals of a Thyroid-Friendly Diet

Hypothyroidism and Hashimoto's thyroiditis are conditions that require careful attention to diet to manage symptoms and support overall health. A thyroid-friendly diet can make a significant difference in how you feel and how well your thyroid functions. In this section, we will explore the key nutrients essential for thyroid health, the foods you should include and avoid, and practical meal planning tips tailored for individuals with hypothyroidism.

Key Nutrients for Thyroid Function

Several nutrients are crucial for the proper functioning of the thyroid gland and the production of thyroid hormones. Understanding these nutrients and ensuring they are included in your diet can help support thyroid health.

1. Iodine: Iodine is a critical component of thyroid hormones. Without sufficient iodine, the thyroid cannot produce enough T3 and T4, leading to hypothyroidism.

Foods rich in iodine include seaweed, iodized salt, fish, dairy products, and eggs. However, it's important to balance iodine intake, as both deficiency and excess can harm thyroid function.

2. Selenium: Selenium is necessary for the conversion of T4 to the more active T3 hormone. It also has antioxidant properties that protect the thyroid gland from oxidative damage. Selenium-rich foods include Brazil nuts, sunflower seeds, fish (like tuna and sardines), and whole grains.

3. Zinc: Zinc plays a role in the synthesis of thyroid hormones and supports the immune system. Good sources of zinc are oysters, beef, chicken, pumpkin seeds, and lentils.

4. Iron: Iron is essential for the production of thyroid hormones and helps maintain healthy red blood cells. Iron deficiency can exacerbate hypothyroidism. Foods rich in iron include red meat, poultry, spinach, lentils, and fortified cereals.

5. Vitamin D: Vitamin D deficiency is common in individuals with thyroid disorders. It supports the immune system and can help reduce inflammation. Sources of

vitamin D include fatty fish, fortified dairy products, and sunlight exposure.

6. Vitamin B12: Hypothyroidism can sometimes lead to low levels of vitamin B12, which is important for energy production and neurological function. Sources of B12 include meat, dairy products, eggs, and fortified plant-based milks.

7. Omega-3 Fatty Acids: Omega-3s have anti-inflammatory properties that can benefit thyroid health. They are found in fatty fish like salmon and mackerel, flaxseeds, chia seeds, and walnuts.

Foods to Include and Avoid

Certain foods can support thyroid function, while others may interfere with it. Here's a detailed list of what to include and what to avoid in a thyroid-friendly diet.

Foods to Include:

1. Seaweed: Rich in iodine, seaweed varieties such as kelp, nori, and wakame can help meet your iodine needs. However, consume them in moderation to avoid excessive iodine intake.

2. Fish and Seafood: Fatty fish like salmon, mackerel, and sardines provide both iodine and omega-3 fatty acids. Shellfish, including shrimp and scallops, are also excellent sources of iodine.

3. Nuts and Seeds: Brazil nuts are particularly high in selenium. Other beneficial nuts and seeds include sunflower seeds, flaxseeds, chia seeds, and walnuts, which provide a variety of essential nutrients.

4. Lean Meats and Poultry: These are good sources of zinc and iron. Choose lean cuts of beef, chicken, and turkey to minimize saturated fat intake.

5. Dairy Products: Milk, yogurt, and cheese provide iodine, vitamin D, and calcium. Opt for low-fat or non-fat versions to manage calorie intake.

6. Whole Grains: Whole grains like quinoa, brown rice, oats, and barley are rich in nutrients like iron and B vitamins. They also provide fiber, which can help with digestive health.

7. Fruits and Vegetables: Berries, leafy greens, and cruciferous vegetables (when cooked) are packed with vitamins, minerals, and antioxidants. Cooking cruciferous vegetables reduces their goitrogenic effects.

8. Legumes: Beans, lentils, and chickpeas are good sources of iron, zinc, and fiber. They can be incorporated into a variety of dishes to enhance nutrient intake.

9. Eggs: Eggs are an excellent source of iodine, selenium, and B vitamins. They are also versatile and can be included in various meals throughout the day.

10. Healthy Fats: Olive oil, avocado, and coconut oil provide healthy fats that support overall health and reduce inflammation.

Foods to Avoid:

1. Gluten: Some individuals with hypothyroidism, particularly those with Hashimoto's thyroiditis, may benefit from a gluten-free diet. Gluten can trigger an autoimmune response in susceptible individuals. Avoid wheat, barley, and rye, and look for gluten-free alternatives.

2. Soy Products: Soy contains compounds that can interfere with thyroid hormone absorption and production. Limit intake of soy milk, tofu, tempeh, and soy-based processed foods.

3. Processed Foods: Highly processed foods often contain unhealthy fats, sugars, and additives that can exacerbate inflammation and interfere with thyroid function. Avoid packaged snacks, sugary cereals, and fast food.

4. Cruciferous Vegetables (Raw): Raw broccoli, cauliflower, cabbage, and Brussels sprouts contain goitrogens that can inhibit iodine uptake. Cooking these vegetables reduces their goitrogenic properties, making them safer to consume in moderation.

5. Certain Nuts: While many nuts are beneficial, peanuts and pine nuts contain goitrogens and should be consumed in moderation.

6. High-Sugar Foods: Excessive sugar intake can lead to weight gain and inflammation. Reduce consumption of sweets, sugary drinks, and desserts.

7. Alcohol: Alcohol can disrupt thyroid hormone levels and impair liver function, which is crucial for hormone

conversion. Limit alcohol consumption or avoid it altogether.

8. Caffeine: Excessive caffeine intake can exacerbate symptoms like anxiety and insomnia. Moderation is key, so consider reducing coffee and caffeinated tea consumption.

Meal Planning Tips for Hypothyroidism

Effective meal planning can make managing hypothyroidism easier and more sustainable. Here are some tips to help you create balanced, nutritious meals that support thyroid health.

1. Plan Ahead: Take some time each week to plan your meals and snacks. This helps ensure you have the necessary ingredients on hand and reduces the temptation to reach for unhealthy options.

2. Batch Cooking: Prepare larger quantities of food and store them in the refrigerator or freezer for quick and easy

meals throughout the week. This is especially helpful for busy days when you don't have time to cook.

3. Balanced Meals: Aim for balanced meals that include a source of protein, healthy fats, and complex carbohydrates. This helps stabilize blood sugar levels and provides sustained energy.

4. Portion Control: Be mindful of portion sizes, especially with higher-calorie foods like nuts, seeds, and healthy fats. Eating in moderation helps maintain a healthy weight.

5. Hydration: Staying hydrated is important for overall health. Drink plenty of water throughout the day, and limit sugary drinks and excessive caffeine.

6. Variety: Incorporate a variety of foods to ensure you get a wide range of nutrients. Different foods provide different vitamins and minerals, which are all important for thyroid health.

7. Smart Substitutions: Make healthier substitutions in your favorite recipes. For example, use Greek yogurt instead of sour cream, or quinoa instead of white rice.

8. Mindful Eating: Pay attention to your body's hunger and fullness cues. Eating mindfully can help prevent overeating and promote better digestion.

9. Consistent Eating Schedule: Try to eat meals at regular intervals to keep your energy levels stable. Skipping meals or irregular eating patterns can disrupt metabolism.

10. Listen to Your Body: Everyone's body is different. Pay attention to how your body responds to certain foods and make adjustments as needed. Keep a food journal to track what works best for you.

By following these guidelines and incorporating the recipes from this cookbook, you can create a thyroid-friendly diet that supports your health and well-being. Remember, the key to managing hypothyroidism through diet is consistency and making informed choices that nourish your body.

Energizing Breakfasts

Breakfast is often called the most important meal of the day, and for those managing hypothyroidism, it's crucial to start the day with nutrient-dense foods that support thyroid health and provide sustained energy. This section explores a variety of breakfast options that can help you feel energized and ready to tackle the day. We will delve into smoothies and shakes for a morning boost, nutritious egg dishes and omelettes, and whole grain and gluten-free breakfast options.

Smoothies and Shakes for a Morning Boost

Smoothies and shakes are an excellent way to pack a lot of nutrients into a convenient, easy-to-digest meal. They can be customized to suit your taste preferences and dietary needs, making them a versatile option for breakfast. Here are some key ingredients to include in your thyroid-friendly smoothies and shakes:

1. Leafy Greens: Spinach, kale, and Swiss chard are rich in vitamins, minerals, and antioxidants. They can be added to smoothies without significantly altering the taste but providing a nutrient boost.

2. Berries: Berries such as blueberries, strawberries, and raspberries are high in antioxidants, vitamins, and fiber. They add natural sweetness and vibrant color to your smoothies.

3. Protein Sources: Protein is essential for muscle repair and energy. Include protein-rich ingredients like Greek yogurt, cottage cheese, or plant-based protein powders.

4. Healthy Fats: Healthy fats help keep you full and support overall health. Add avocados, chia seeds, flaxseeds, or a spoonful of nut butter to your smoothies.

5. Liquid Base: Choose a liquid base that complements the flavors and adds additional nutrients. Options include almond milk, coconut milk, unsweetened green tea, or water.

6. Superfoods: Boost the nutritional profile of your smoothies with superfoods like spirulina, maca powder, or acai powder. These can provide additional vitamins, minerals, and antioxidants.

Here are a couple of smoothie recipes to get you started:

Green Goddess Smoothie:

1. 1 cup unsweetened almond milk

2. 1 cup fresh spinach

3. 1/2 cup frozen mango chunks

4. 1/2 avocado

5. 1 tablespoon chia seeds

6. 1 scoop vanilla protein powder

7. Ice cubes (optional)

Blend all ingredients until smooth and creamy. Enjoy a refreshing and nutrient-packed start to your day.

Berry Bliss Shake:
1. 1 cup coconut water

2. 1/2 cup frozen mixed berries

3. 1/2 banana

4. 1/4 cup Greek yogurt

5. 1 tablespoon flaxseeds

6. 1 teaspoon honey (optional)

Blend until smooth and enjoy the delicious, antioxidant-rich shake.

Nutritious Egg Dishes and Omelettes

Eggs are a versatile and nutritious breakfast option that provides high-quality protein, vitamins, and minerals. They can be prepared in numerous ways to keep your breakfast routine exciting and satisfying. Here are some delicious and thyroid-friendly egg dishes and omelettes:

1. Veggie-Packed Omelette: An omelette is a great way to incorporate a variety of vegetables into your breakfast. Vegetables provide fiber, vitamins, and minerals that support thyroid health.

Ingredients:
1. 3 large eggs
2. 1/4 cup chopped bell peppers
3. 1/4 cup chopped tomatoes
4. 1/4 cup chopped spinach
5. 1/4 cup chopped onions
6. 1/4 cup shredded cheese (optional)
7. Salt and pepper to taste

8. 1 tablespoon olive oil

Instructions:

1. Whisk the eggs in a bowl and season with salt and pepper.

2. Heat olive oil in a non-stick skillet over medium heat.

3. Add the chopped vegetables to the skillet and sauté until tender.

4. Pour the eggs over the vegetables and cook until the eggs are set.

5. Sprinkle with cheese if desired and fold the omelette in half.

6. Serve hot and enjoy a nutritious start to your day.

2. Egg Muffins: Egg muffins are perfect for meal prep and can be customized with your favorite ingredients. They are convenient, portable, and make a great on-the-go breakfast.

Ingredients:

1. 6 large eggs

2. 1/4 cup milk (dairy or non-dairy)

3. 1/2 cup chopped vegetables (e.g., spinach, bell peppers, mushrooms)

4. 1/4 cup cooked and crumbled turkey sausage or bacon (optional)

5. 1/4 cup shredded cheese (optional)

6. Salt and pepper to taste

Instructions:

1. Preheat the oven to 350°F (175°C) and grease a muffin tin.

2. In a bowl, whisk the eggs and milk together. Season with salt and pepper.

3. Add the chopped vegetables and cooked meat (if using) to the egg mixture.

4. Pour the mixture into the muffin tin, filling each cup about three-quarters full.

5. Sprinkle with cheese if desired.

6. Bake for 20-25 minutes, or until the eggs are set and lightly golden.

7. Allow to cool slightly before removing from the tin. Store in the refrigerator for up to 5 days.

3. Shakshuka: Shakshuka is a flavorful Middle Eastern dish that features poached eggs in a spicy tomato sauce. It's a hearty and satisfying breakfast that can be enjoyed with a side of whole grain bread or gluten-free toast.

Ingredients:

1. 1 tablespoon olive oil

2. 1 onion, chopped

3. 1 red bell pepper, chopped

4. 3 cloves garlic, minced

5. 1 can (14 oz) diced tomatoes

6. 1 teaspoon cumin

7. 1 teaspoon paprika

8. 1/2 teaspoon chili powder

9. Salt and pepper to taste

10. 4-6 large eggs

11. Fresh cilantro or parsley for garnish

Instructions:

1. Heat olive oil in a large skillet over medium heat. Add the onion and bell pepper, cooking until softened.

2. Add the garlic and cook for another minute.

3. Stir in the diced tomatoes and spices. Simmer for 10 minutes until the sauce thickens.

4. Make small wells in the sauce and crack an egg into each well.

5. Cover the skillet and cook until the eggs are set to your liking.

6. Garnish with fresh herbs and serve hot.

Whole Grain and Gluten-Free Breakfast Options

For those with hypothyroidism, especially those sensitive to gluten, whole grain and gluten-free breakfast options can provide essential nutrients without causing digestive issues. Here are some wholesome and delicious choices:

1. Quinoa Breakfast Bowl: Quinoa is a complete protein and provides essential amino acids, fiber, and minerals. It's a versatile grain that can be used in both sweet and savory breakfast dishes.

Ingredients:

1. 1 cup cooked quinoa

2. 1/2 cup almond milk

3. 1/2 teaspoon cinnamon

4. 1 tablespoon honey or maple syrup

5. 1/4 cup fresh berries

6. 1 tablespoon chopped nuts (e.g., almonds, walnuts)

Instructions:

1. In a small saucepan, warm the cooked quinoa and almond milk over medium heat.

2. Stir in the cinnamon and honey or maple syrup.

3. Serve topped with fresh berries and chopped nuts for a nutritious and satisfying breakfast.

2. Gluten-Free Oatmeal: Oatmeal is a comforting and filling breakfast option that can be easily made gluten-free by using certified gluten-free oats. It's rich in fiber and can be customized with various toppings.

Ingredients:

1. 1 cup gluten-free rolled oats

2. 2 cups water or almond milk

3. 1/2 teaspoon cinnamon

4. 1 tablespoon chia seeds

5. 1/4 cup fresh fruit (e.g., bananas, berries, apples)

6. 1 tablespoon nut butter or seeds (e.g., almond butter, sunflower seeds)

Instructions:

1. In a saucepan, bring the water or almond milk to a boil.

2. Add the oats and reduce the heat to a simmer. Cook for about 5 minutes, stirring occasionally.

3. Stir in the cinnamon and chia seeds.

4. Serve topped with fresh fruit and nut butter or seeds for added flavor and nutrients.

3. Chia Seed Pudding: Chia seeds are a powerhouse of nutrients, including omega-3 fatty acids, fiber, and protein. Chia seed pudding is a convenient make-ahead breakfast that can be customized with your favorite flavors.

Ingredients:

1. 1/4 cup chia seeds

2. 1 cup almond milk

3. 1 tablespoon honey or maple syrup

4. 1/2 teaspoon vanilla extract

5. Fresh fruit or nuts for topping

Instructions:

1. In a bowl, whisk together the chia seeds, almond milk, honey or maple syrup, and vanilla extract.

2. Cover and refrigerate for at least 4 hours, or overnight, until the mixture thickens.

3. Stir well before serving and top with fresh fruit or nuts.

4. Sweet Potato Hash: Sweet potatoes are rich in vitamins, minerals, and fiber. A sweet potato hash makes a hearty and satisfying breakfast that can be paired with eggs or enjoyed on its own.

Ingredients:

1. 1 large sweet potato, peeled and diced

2. 1 tablespoon olive oil

3. 1/2 onion, chopped

4. 1 red bell pepper, chopped

5. 1 teaspoon smoked paprika

6. Salt and pepper to taste

7. Fresh herbs for garnish

Instructions:

1. Heat olive oil in a large skillet over medium heat.

2. Add the sweet potato and cook for about 10 minutes, until tender.

3. Add the onion and bell pepper, cooking until softened.

4. Stir in the smoked paprika, salt, and pepper.

5. Cook until the vegetables are fully cooked and slightly crispy.

6. Garnish with fresh herbs and serve hot.

Balanced Lunches

A balanced lunch is essential for maintaining energy levels and supporting thyroid health throughout the day. Here, we will explore hearty salads with thyroid-supporting ingredients, protein-packed sandwiches and wraps, and nourishing soups and stews. Each of these options offers a variety of nutrients to help manage hypothyroidism and promote overall well-being.

Hearty Salads with Thyroid-Supporting Ingredients

Salads can be a powerhouse of nutrients when they are made with the right ingredients. For a thyroid-friendly salad, focus on incorporating a mix of colorful vegetables, lean proteins, healthy fats, and thyroid-supporting foods.

1. Mixed Greens and Salmon Salad: Start with a base of mixed greens such as spinach, kale, and arugula, which are rich in vitamins and minerals. Add a serving of grilled or baked salmon for a boost of omega-3 fatty acids and selenium, both of which are beneficial for thyroid function. Toss in some cherry tomatoes, cucumbers, and red bell peppers for added vitamins and antioxidants. Finish with a dressing made from olive oil, lemon juice, and a touch of Dijon mustard.

2. Quinoa and Avocado Salad: Quinoa is a complete protein and provides essential amino acids and fiber.

Combine cooked quinoa with diced avocado, which is rich in healthy fats and supports hormone production. Add black beans, corn, red onion, and cilantro for a southwestern flair. Dress with a lime vinaigrette made from lime juice, olive oil, and cumin.

3. Roasted Beet and Goat Cheese Salad: Roasted beets are rich in antioxidants and fiber, which can aid in digestion. Pair them with creamy goat cheese for a delightful texture contrast. Add mixed greens, walnuts (for omega-3s), and sliced apples for sweetness. Drizzle with a balsamic reduction for a touch of acidity and flavor.

Protein-Packed Sandwiches and Wraps

Sandwiches and wraps are convenient lunch options that can be packed with protein to keep you full and satisfied.

1. Turkey and Avocado Wrap: Use a whole-grain or gluten-free wrap and fill it with sliced turkey breast, which is a lean source of protein. Add avocado for healthy fats, spinach for iron and vitamins, and sliced tomatoes for a

juicy, fresh element. A smear of hummus adds flavor and additional protein.

2. Grilled Chicken and Veggie Sandwich: Choose a whole-grain or gluten-free bread and layer it with grilled chicken breast, which provides lean protein. Add a mix of roasted vegetables such as bell peppers, zucchini, and eggplant for a hearty and nutritious filling. Spread a little pesto or Greek yogurt for added flavor and creaminess.

3. Egg Salad Lettuce Wraps: For a low-carb option, make an egg salad using hard-boiled eggs, Greek yogurt, a touch of mustard, and chopped celery. Serve the egg salad in large lettuce leaves (such as romaine or iceberg) for a crunchy and refreshing wrap.

Nourishing Soups and Stews

Soups and stews are comforting and can be made in large batches for easy meal prep. They are perfect for incorporating a variety of thyroid-supporting ingredients.

1. Lentil and Spinach Soup: Lentils are high in protein and fiber, making them a filling base for soup. Add spinach for

iron and vitamins, carrots, celery, and onions for additional nutrients. Season with garlic, cumin, and turmeric for a flavorful and anti-inflammatory boost.

2. Chicken and Vegetable Stew: A hearty chicken stew can be packed with vegetables like carrots, potatoes, celery, and peas. Use bone-in chicken thighs for added flavor and nutrients. Simmer with herbs like thyme and rosemary for a fragrant and nutritious meal.

3. Butternut Squash and Ginger Soup: Butternut squash is rich in vitamins A and C and provides a creamy texture when blended. Add fresh ginger for its anti-inflammatory properties and a touch of spice. Garnish with a dollop of Greek yogurt and a sprinkle of pumpkin seeds for added protein and crunch.

Satisfying Dinners

Dinner is an important meal that provides the nutrients and energy needed to support your body's functions and promote restful sleep. For those managing hypothyroidism, choosing the right dinner options can help balance hormones and improve overall health. In this section, we will explore lean protein entrees, thyroid-friendly fish and seafood dishes, and vegetarian and vegan dinner ideas.

Lean Protein Entrees

Lean proteins are essential for muscle repair and growth, and they can help keep you feeling full without adding excessive calories or unhealthy fats.

1. Grilled Chicken with Roasted Vegetables: Grilled chicken breast is an excellent source of lean protein. Marinate the chicken in olive oil, lemon juice, garlic, and herbs like rosemary and thyme for added flavor. Serve with a side of roasted vegetables such as Brussels sprouts, carrots, and sweet potatoes, which provide fiber, vitamins, and minerals.

2. Turkey Meatballs with Zucchini Noodles: Turkey is a lean protein that can be transformed into delicious meatballs. Mix ground turkey with garlic, onions, parsley, and a touch of Parmesan cheese. Bake the meatballs until golden brown. Serve with zucchini noodles (zoodles)

tossed in marinara sauce for a low-carb, nutrient-dense alternative to traditional pasta.

3. Baked Pork Tenderloin with Apple Chutney: Pork tenderloin is another lean protein option. Season it with a mix of paprika, garlic powder, and thyme, then bake until tender. Serve with a homemade apple chutney made from diced apples, onions, apple cider vinegar, and a touch of honey for a sweet and savory combination.

Thyroid-Friendly Fish and Seafood Dishes

Fish and seafood are rich in omega-3 fatty acids, iodine, and selenium, all of which are crucial for thyroid health.

1. Baked Salmon with Quinoa and Asparagus: Salmon is a top choice for thyroid support due to its high omega-3 and selenium content. Bake a salmon fillet with a drizzle of olive oil, lemon slices, and fresh dill. Serve with a side of quinoa, which provides complete protein and fiber, and steamed asparagus for added vitamins and minerals.

2. Shrimp Stir-Fry with Broccoli and Bell Peppers: Shrimp is low in calories but high in iodine and protein. Sauté shrimp with fresh garlic and ginger, then add broccoli and bell peppers for a colorful and nutrient-packed dish. Serve over brown rice or cauliflower rice for a satisfying meal.

3. Cod with Tomato Basil Sauce: Cod is a mild white fish that pairs well with a variety of flavors. Bake cod fillets with a sauce made from tomatoes, fresh basil, garlic, and olive oil. This dish is light yet packed with essential nutrients that support thyroid function.

Vegetarian and Vegan Dinner Ideas

Vegetarian and vegan meals can be just as satisfying and are excellent for incorporating a variety of thyroid-supporting vegetables and plant-based proteins.

1. Chickpea and Spinach Curry: Chickpeas are rich in protein and fiber, making them a hearty base for a vegetarian curry. Sauté onions, garlic, and ginger, then add canned chickpeas, spinach, and a blend of spices like turmeric, cumin, and coriander. Simmer with coconut milk

for a creamy and flavorful dish. Serve with brown rice or quinoa.

2. Lentil Shepherd's Pie: Lentils are a great source of plant-based protein and can replace meat in this classic dish. Cook lentils with onions, carrots, celery, and thyme, then top with mashed sweet potatoes. Bake until golden brown for a comforting and nutrient-dense meal.

3. Stuffed Bell Peppers with Quinoa and Black Beans: Bell peppers are loaded with vitamins A and C. Stuff them with a mixture of cooked quinoa, black beans, corn, tomatoes, and spices like cumin and chili powder. Bake until the peppers are tender and serve with a side salad for a complete meal.

Desserts and Sweet Treats

Desserts can still be enjoyed while managing hypothyroidism by choosing recipes that are low in sugar, incorporate nutritious fruits, and provide indulgence without compromising health. Here are some ideas for creating delicious desserts and sweet treats that support thyroid health and align with your dietary goals.

Low-Sugar Baking Recipes

Reducing sugar intake is beneficial for overall health, including thyroid function. Here are some low-sugar baking recipes that satisfy your sweet tooth without causing spikes in blood sugar:

1. Almond Flour Banana Bread: Almond flour is a nutritious alternative to traditional flour, providing protein, healthy fats, and fiber. Combine almond flour with ripe bananas, eggs, a touch of honey or maple syrup, and cinnamon. Bake until golden brown for a moist and flavorful banana bread that's naturally sweet.

2. Oatmeal Raisin Cookies: Oats are high in fiber and can help stabilize blood sugar levels. Make oatmeal raisin cookies using rolled oats, raisins, cinnamon, and a small amount of coconut sugar or stevia for sweetness. These cookies are chewy, satisfying, and lower in sugar compared to traditional recipes.

3. Dark Chocolate Avocado Mousse: Avocado adds a creamy texture and healthy fats to desserts. Blend ripe avocados with unsweetened cocoa powder, a splash of vanilla extract, and a small amount of honey or agave syrup. Chill until firm for a decadent chocolate mousse that's rich in antioxidants and good fats.

Delicious Fruit-Based Desserts

Fruits are naturally sweet and packed with vitamins, minerals, and fiber. Here are some fruit-based desserts that are refreshing and nutritious:

1. Mixed Berry Parfait: Layer fresh berries (such as strawberries, blueberries, and raspberries) with Greek yogurt or coconut yogurt in a glass. Top with a sprinkle of granola or crushed nuts for added crunch and protein. This parfait is a balanced dessert option that satisfies sweet cravings while providing essential nutrients.

2. Grilled Pineapple with Cinnamon: Grilling pineapple caramelizes its natural sugars and enhances its sweetness. Sprinkle pineapple slices with cinnamon before grilling

until golden brown. Serve warm as a simple yet satisfying dessert or snack.

3. Frozen Banana Pops: Peel bananas and cut them in half. Insert a popsicle stick into each half, then dip them in melted dark chocolate. Roll in chopped nuts or shredded coconut and freeze until solid. These banana pops are a fun and guilt-free treat that combines fruit, chocolate, and crunchy toppings.

Indulgent Yet Healthy Sweets

It's possible to indulge in sweets occasionally while still supporting your thyroid health. Here are some ideas for healthier versions of classic indulgent desserts:

1. Chia Seed Pudding with Fresh Berries: Chia seeds are rich in fiber and omega-3 fatty acids. Mix chia seeds with almond milk, a touch of vanilla extract, and a small amount of honey or maple syrup. Let it sit overnight in the refrigerator until it thickens. Serve topped with fresh berries for a nutritious and satisfying pudding.

2. Greek Yogurt Cheesecake Bars: Use Greek yogurt as a base for cheesecake bars instead of cream cheese. Mix Greek yogurt with a little honey or stevia, lemon juice, and vanilla extract. Pour over a nut or oat crust and bake until set. Chill in the refrigerator before slicing into bars. These cheesecake bars are creamy, tangy, and lower in fat compared to traditional recipes.

3. Baked Apples with Cinnamon and Walnuts: Core apples and stuff them with a mixture of chopped walnuts, cinnamon, and a touch of honey. Bake until the apples are tender and serve warm. Baked apples are naturally sweet and comforting, making them a satisfying dessert option.

Managing Hypothyroidism with Lifestyle Changes

Managing hypothyroidism involves more than just dietary adjustments; incorporating lifestyle changes can significantly impact thyroid health and overall well-being. Here are key lifestyle strategies including exercise recommendations, stress management techniques, and the importance of sleep in supporting thyroid function.

Exercise and Physical Activity Recommendations

Regular exercise is beneficial for individuals with hypothyroidism as it can help boost metabolism, improve mood, and promote overall health. Here are some exercise recommendations tailored for managing hypothyroidism:

1. Aerobic Exercise: Engage in moderate-intensity aerobic activities such as brisk walking, cycling, swimming, or dancing for at least 150 minutes per week, as recommended by health guidelines. Aerobic exercise helps stimulate thyroid hormone production and can aid in weight management, which is often a concern for individuals with hypothyroidism.

2. Strength Training: Incorporate strength training exercises using resistance bands, free weights, or bodyweight exercises (like squats, lunges, and push-ups) at least twice a

week. Building muscle mass can help increase metabolism and support overall strength and stamina.

3. Yoga and Stretching: Practicing yoga or stretching exercises can help improve flexibility, reduce muscle stiffness, and alleviate stress, which is beneficial for thyroid health. Certain yoga poses, such as shoulder stands and fish pose, are believed to stimulate the thyroid gland.

4. Interval Training: Consider incorporating interval training, alternating between periods of high-intensity exercise and recovery periods. This type of workout can help increase cardiovascular fitness and metabolic rate.

Stress Management Techniques

Chronic stress can negatively impact thyroid function and exacerbate symptoms of hypothyroidism. Implementing stress management techniques can help support thyroid health and overall well-being:

1. Mindfulness and Meditation: Practice mindfulness meditation or deep-breathing exercises to reduce stress levels and promote relaxation. These techniques can help

lower cortisol levels, which can interfere with thyroid hormone production.

2. Yoga and Tai Chi: Engage in mind-body practices like yoga or tai chi, which combine movement with meditation and breathing exercises. These practices can help reduce stress, improve mood, and enhance overall mental and physical well-being.

3. Time Management: Effective time management strategies can help reduce feelings of overwhelm and stress. Prioritize tasks, set realistic goals, and delegate responsibilities when possible to create a balanced lifestyle.

4. Social Support: Maintain strong social connections with friends, family, or support groups. Talking with others who understand your condition can provide emotional support and reduce feelings of isolation.

Sleep and Its Impact on Thyroid Health

Quality sleep is crucial for maintaining optimal thyroid function and overall health. Poor sleep habits can disrupt hormone production and exacerbate symptoms of hypothyroidism. Here's how to improve sleep quality:

1. Establish a Sleep Routine: Maintain a consistent sleep schedule by going to bed and waking up at the same time each day, even on weekends. This helps regulate your body's internal clock and promote better sleep.

2. Create a Relaxing Sleep Environment: Make your bedroom conducive to sleep by keeping it cool, dark, and quiet. Use blackout curtains, earplugs, or a white noise machine if needed to block out distractions.

3. Limit Screen Time: Avoid electronic devices such as smartphones, tablets, and computers at least an hour before bedtime. The blue light emitted from screens can interfere with the production of melatonin, a hormone that regulates sleep.

4. Practice Relaxation Techniques: Wind down before bed with calming activities such as reading a book, taking a warm bath, or practicing gentle yoga stretches. These activities signal to your body that it's time to relax and prepare for sleep.

5. Limit Caffeine and Alcohol: Reduce consumption of caffeine and alcohol, especially in the hours leading up to bedtime. These substances can disrupt sleep patterns and decrease sleep quality.

Hypothyroidism Diet Recipes

Beef Stir-Fry with Vegetables

Ingredients:

1. 1 red paprika

2. 1 yellow paprika

3. 1 green paprika

4. 3 carrots

5. 5 scallions

6. 200 grams fresh mung bean sprouts

7. 1 red chili pepper

8. 600 grams beef fillet

9. 1 pc fresh ginger (about 1.5 cm)

10. 2 tbsps sesame oil

11. 2 tbsps coarsely chopped parsley

12. Soy sauce (to taste)

13. Freshly ground peppers

Preparation steps

1. Rinse the bell peppers, cut in half, remove seeds and white membrane and cut flesh into thin strips. Peel the

carrots and cut into thin sticks. Rinse, trim and slice the scallions diagonally. Rinse the mung bean sprouts in a colander and drain well. Rinse the chile pepper, cut in half, remove seeds and finely chop.

2. Rinse the beef, pat dry and cut into strips. Peel the ginger and finely grate. Heat oil in a wok and brown the beef strips on all sides. Remove from the wok and set aside.

3. Add the vegetables, ginger, parsley and chile pepper to the wok and stir-fry until browned, stirring constantly. Return the beef to the wok and stir to combine. Serve seasoned with soy sauce and pepper to taste.

Raspberry Cream Gels

INGREDIENTS

1. 6 ounces fresh raspberries (about 1 1/2 cups)

2. 1/2 cup water, divided

3. 2 tablespoons plus 1 teaspoon maple syrup

4. Pinch sea salt

5. 1/2 teaspoon vanilla extract

6. 1 tablespoon plus 2 teaspoons unflavored gelatin

7. 1 teaspoon lemon juice

8. 1/4 cup plain dairy-free yogurt

9. Optional equipment: Heart-shaped Silicone Mold

INSTRUCTIONS

1. In a small saucepan combine raspberries, 1/4 cup water, maple syrup, salt, and vanilla. Use a potato masher to mash the berries. Bring to a boil over medium-high heat. Let bubble for 5 minutes.

2. Meanwhile, place the remaining 1/4 cup water (cool or cold) in a bowl. Sprinkle the gelatin powder evenly across the top of the water and let sit 5 minutes. This is called "blooming" the gelatin and will prevent lumps. It will look wrinkly and weird-- that's normal

3. When raspberry mixture is done cooking, strain it into a medium mixing bowl through a fine mesh sieve. Use a rubber spatula to press out the juice (while straining out the seeds).

4. Return strained raspberry mixture to small saucepan and stir in bloomed gelatin. Whisk until gelatin is dissolved and no visible granules remain. The mixture needs to be warm for this to happen, so if it has cooled off, you may need to reheat the mixture over low heat. Note: Avoid boiling the

gelatin or getting it hotter than 140 F, or it may lose its gelling power.

5. Once gelatin is dissolved, add lemon juice and yogurt, and whisk to combine until no lumps remain.

6. Pour mixture into a heart-shaped silicone mold if desired, or into a small pyrex dish (approx. 5 x 7 inches, or similar). Let chill for at least 4 hours or until completely set. Remove from mold or cut into bite-sized pieces and enjoy.

Redcurrant Muffins with Meringue Topping

Ingredients

For the redcurrant puree:

1. 2 cups red currant

2. ⅛ cup water

3. ¼ cup powdered sugar

For the cupcakes:

1. 1 ½ cups all-purpose flour

2. 2 tsps baking powder

3. ⅔ cup superfine caster sugar

4. 2 eggs (separated)

5. 8 tbsps sunflower oil

6. 6 tbsps milk

7. ½ unwaxed lemon (juice and finely grated zest)

8. 1 ½ cups red currant

For the meringue:

1. 2 egg whites

2. ½ cup superfine caster sugar

Preparation steps

1. For the redcurrant puree: put the redcurrants and water in a pan. Bring to a simmer and cook for 5-10 minutes, until soft and pulpy.

2. Rub through a sieve, to remove the skins and pips, and while still warm sift in the icing sugar and stir to dissolve. Set aside to cool completely.

3. For the cupcakes: heat the oven to 180°C (160° fan) 350°F gas 4. Place paper cases in a 10 hole muffin tin.

4. Sift the flour and baking powder into a mixing bowl.

5. Whisk together the sugar, egg yolks, oil, milk, lemon juice and zest until smooth. Stir into the flour until blended.

6. Spoon into the paper cases and bake for 15-20 minutes until golden and risen. Leave in the tin.

7. For the meringue: whisk the egg whites until they stand in soft peaks. Gradually whisk in the sugar until the mixture is stiff. Add 3 tablespoons of the fruit puree and gently swirl it through to marble.

8. Spread any remaining fruit puree on top of the cakes.

9. Spoon the meringue on top of the cupcakes. Return the cupcakes to the oven for 5-7 minutes, until the meringue is set. Place the cakes on a wire rack to cool completely.

BUTTER CHICKEN WITH VEGETABLES THYROID AUTOIMMUNE MEAL PLAN

Equipment
1. slow cooker

Ingredients
1. 2 onions, diced
2. 3 cloves garlic, minced
3. 3 tbsp butter
4. 2 tbsp fresh ginger, grated

5. 2 tsp chili powder (optional depending on heat level of your chili powder)

6. 1/4 tsp ground coriander

7. 1/4 tsp turmeric

8. 1/2 tsp cinnamon

9. 1/2 tsp ground cumin

10. Salt and pepper to taste

11. 1 28 oz can diced tomatoes

12. 1 cup chicken broth

13. 1/4 cup almond butter

14. 3 lbs boneless, skinless chicken breast, cubed

15. 2 tbsp fresh cilantro, finely chopped

16. 2 potatoes, chopped into 1 inch pieces

17. 1/2 small squash, chopped into 1 inch pieces

Instructions

1. Place potatoes and squash on bottom of crock pot.

2. In a medium bowl, combine onions, garlic, butter, ginger, chili powder, coriander, turmeric, cinnamon, cumin, salt, pepper and tomatoes.

3. Mix together and add to slow cooker.

4. In a separate small bowl, whisk together the almond butter and chicken broth.

5. Once mixed, pour into the slow cooker slowly, while continually whisking.

6. Add chicken.

7. Cook on low for anywhere from 5 to 8 hours.

8. Remove chicken, potatoes and squash when they are done and reserve the sauce in the crock pot.

9. Using a hand blender, puree the sauce until smooth (do not have to remove the sauce fromthe slow cooker to do this).

10. Sprinkle with fresh coriander before serving.

Paleo Pumpkin Muffins with Chocolate Chips

Ingredients

1. 2½ cups almond flour

2. ¼ cup coconut sugar

3. ¼ cup ground flaxseeds

4. 1 teaspoon baking soda

5. ½ teaspoon ground cinnamon

6. ½ teaspoon sea salt

7. 3 large eggs

8. ¼ cup unsweetened pumpkin puree

9. 2 tablespoons pure maple syrup or local honey

10. ½ teaspoon vanilla extract

11. ½ cup dairy-free dark chocolate chips

Instructions

1. Preheat oven to 375°F. Line a muffin tin with paper muffin cups liners.

2. Mix dry ingredients (flour, sugar, flaxseeds, baking soda, cinnamon, and salt) together in a large bowl with a whisk or a fork. Ensure that any lumps in the flour are broken up.

3. In a separate bowl, whisk eggs, pumpkin puree, maple syrup or honey, and vanilla together until well combined.

4. Combine the wet and dry mixtures and stir with a rubber spatula until well mixed. Gently fold in chocolate chips, taking care to avoid over-mixing. Batter will be thicker than most muffin batters, but will be spoonable.

5. Spoon batter into muffin cups until approximately ¾ full. Place muffin tin in the oven and bake for 20-22 minutes, until tops are golden. Test doneness by inserting a

toothpick into the center of a muffin. If it comes out clean, the muffins are done.

QUINOA SALAD WITH ROASTED VEGETABLES

Ingredients

1. 4 cups chicken stock

2. 2 cups quinoa, soaked overnight in water and 1 tablespoon vinegar and drained

3. 1 medium zucchini, cut into 1/4-inch thick slices

4. 2 medium carrots, cut into 1/4-inch thick slices

5. 1 medium red onion, cut into 1/4-inch thick slices

6. 1 red bell pepper, cut into 1/4-inch thick slices

7. 3 tablespoons coconut oil

8. Sea salt and freshly ground black pepper

9. 1 tablespoon tomato paste

10. 1/4 cup fresh lemon juice

11. 3/4 teaspoon coarse sea salt

Instructions

1. Preheat oven to 400°F and adjust rack to middle position. Bring stock to a boil in a large sauce pan. Pour in quinoa and bring to a boil. Lower heat to low and cover with a lid. Cook until quinoa is soft and stock has been absorbed, about 15-20 minutes.

2. Place vegetables on a large baking sheet and toss with coconut oil. Season with salt and pepper.

3. Roast vegetables in oven until edges are golden, about 30 minutes, stirring half way through roasting. Cool. Pour the quinoa in a large bowl. In a small bowl whisk together tomato paste and lemon juice. Pour mixture over quinoa and stir until incorporated. Add vegetables and salt and stir. Serve at room temperature.

Loaded Mediterranean Salmon

INGREDIENTS

1. 2 pounds wild salmon filet, skin removed

2. ½ tsp fine sea salt, or to taste

3. ¼ tsp Freshly ground pepper

4. ¼ tsp Paprika

5. ¼ tsp Ground Ginger

6. ¼ tsp Dried Dill

7. bulb fresh fennel, thinly sliced

8. 1 cup artichoke hearts, quartered

9. 1 cup fresh tomatoes, diced

10. 1/2 cup kalamata olives, sliced

11. 1/3 cup capers, drained

12. 1/2 cup Dairy-free Lemon Basil Pesto (or your favorite pesto)

13. 1 lemon, cut into wedges

INSTRUCTIONS

1. Preheat oven to 400 F.

2. Cut the salmon fillet into serving-size pieces and arrange skin-side-down in either a large, oven-safe skillet (with lid), or a 9 x 13-inch glass baking dish.

3. Lightly sprinkle the salmon with salt, pepper, paprika, ginger, and dill.

4. Top the salmon with remaining ingredients, dropping the pesto on in small dollops.

5. Cover pan with oven-safe lid, or cover baking dish tightly with foil, and place on center rack of oven for 20 minutes.

6. Remove fish from oven and let rest, covered, for 5 minutes to finish cooking.

7. Remove lid/cover, and use a fork to check fish for doneness in the thickest part of the filet. If necessary, return to oven for 5 to 10 additional minutes.

8. Serve with lemon wedges and cauliflower rice or basmati rice to soak up some of the wonderful cooking juices. Optionally, you might add a small pinch of saffron threads to the rice, which is a lovely compliment. Enjoy!

Chinese Egg Noodles with Vegetables

Ingredients

1. 2 small bok choy

2. 1 large paprika (red)

3. 300 grams bamboo shoots (sliced)

4. 300 grams shiitake mushrooms

5. 1 pc ginger (2 cm)

6. 1 garlic clove

7. 1 chili pepper (red)

8. 8 small potatoes (cooked the previous day)

9. 6 tbsps peanut oil

10. 300 grams chinese egg noodle

For seasoning:

1. 3 tbsps water

2. 1 tbsp sugar

3. 4 tbsps rice wine

4. 5 tbsps soy sauce

5. 3 tbsps oyster sauce

6. 2 tbsps sesame seeds

Preparation steps

1. Soak the Chinese egg noodles in cold water.

2. Cut the stalk from the Pak Choi and divide into individual leaves. Rinse and shake dry. Drain and rinse the bamboo shoots. Clean the shiitake mushrooms with a paper towel and remove the stems. Cut the potatoes into quarters.

3. Rinse the chile pepper and cut lengthwise. Remove the seeds and the white inner skin. Chop finely. Peel the garlic cloves and dice finely. Peel the ginger and grate finely.

4. Heat 1 tablespoon oil in a wok and sauté the chile pepper, garlic and ginger for 1-2 minutes. Transfer to a plate and keep in a preheated oven at 100°C (approximately 160°F). Cook the other ingredients one at a time in 1

tablespoon the oil. Cook each for 4-6 minutes. Stirring constantly and sprinkle each with 1-2 tablespoons of seasoning sauce. Transfer to the plate and keep warm.

5. When all the vegetables are cooked, pour 500 ml (approximately 2 cups) of water into the wok and bring to a boil. Drain the Chinese noodles and add to the boiling water. Cook for about 3-5 minutes until tender according to package label.

6. Drain the pasta and put into 4 bowls. Sprinkle with the remaining seasoning sauce and arrange the vegetables on top. Sprinkle with the sesame, garlic, chilli and ginger mixture. Serve hot.

Thyroid-Friendly Mediterranean Juice

Ingredients

1. 1 red pepper, seeded

2. 1 tomato

3. 1 lemon, peeled (optional)

4. 1 cucumber

5. 4 sprigs oregano

6. Pinch sea salt (optional)

Directions

1. Wash all produce well

2. Cut off stem of red pepper and remove seeds

3. Peel lemon if desired, or if the lemon isn't organic

4. Slice cucumber and tomato to fit your juicer

5. Juice all ingredients, wrapping oregano around cucumber to get best yield. Juice stems with oregano for maximum flavor.

6. Garnish with oregano leaves, lemon slice and pinch of Himalayan or sea salt.

Thai Peanut Chicken Skewers

INGREDIENTS

1. 1 ½ lbs boneless, skinless chicken breasts (preferably pasture-raised), cut into bite-sized chunks

2. Wooden skewers, soaked in water for 30 minutes before putting chicken on them

Marinade:

3. 3 tablespoons coconut aminos (or sub. tamari)

4. 2 tablespoons honey

5. 1 tablespoon toasted sesame oil

6. Juice from a lime

7. 2 garlic cloves, minced or 1 tablespoon minced garlic

8. 1 teaspoon Sriracha or hot pepper sauce

9. ⅛ teaspoon red pepper flakes

Peanut Sauce:

1. 2 tablespoons powdered peanut butter or about 1 1/2 tablespoons natural peanut butter, or to taste

2. 1 tablespoon coconut aminos (or sub. tamari)

3. 1 tablespoon water

4. ⅛ teaspoon garlic powder

5. ¼ teaspoon black pepper

6. ⅛ teaspoon sriracha

7. 1 teaspoon coconut sugar (or sub. brown sugar)

8. ⅛ teaspoon toasted sesame oil

INSTRUCTIONS

1. In a medium mixing bowl, combine all the marinade ingredients. Add the cut chicken and toss to coat. Marinate for at least 3-4 hours or overnight.

2. To make the peanut sauce, combine all ingredients and whisk until well combined.

3. Preheat grill until hot. Thread chicken evenly onto skewers. Place the skewers on the grill over low heat. Cooking times may vary but cook chicken while flipping them until cooked through, 5 to 7 minutes per side.

4. Serve skewers with peanut sauce for dipping.

Cauliflower with Ginger

Ingredients

1. 1 sml/med Cauliflower head

2. 4 Tbsp Coconut oil

3. 1 tsp Coriander seeds

4. 1 1/2 Tbsp Ginger freshly minced

5. 1 Green chili seeded and chopped

6. 1 tsp Turmeric

7. 1/2 tsp Celtic sea salt

8. 2 tsp Lemon Juice freshly squeezed

9. 2 Tbsp Coriander chopped fresh

Instructions

1. Separate cauliflower into florets, wash well and drain.

2. Heat 3 tablespoons of oil over high heat in a fry pan.

3. When very hot, add the coriander seed and fry for 10 seconds. Add in the ginger, chilies and stir for a couple of seconds. Immediately add turmeric and salt, following with straight away with the cauliflower.

4. Stir rapidly to prevent burning and to distribute the spices.

5. Add 1/4 cup of hot water, reduce the heat to medium - low, cover and cook for 20 to 25 minutes, stirring once or twice.

6. Increase the heat to medium, uncover and stir fry to evaporate remaining moisture and to lightly brown the cauliflower, 5 to 10 minutes stirring carefully.

7. If vegetable look a little dry, stir in the rest of the oil. Add lemon juice and the coriander leaves and toss through.

8. Serve immediately as a side dish.

HONEY MUSTARD CHICKEN SALAD

INGREDIENTS

FOR THE MARINADE:

1. 4 chicken breasts

2. 1/4 cup fresh lemon juice

3. 1/4 cup extra virgin olive oil

4. 3 cloves garlic, minced

5. 1 teaspoon Celtic Sea Salt

FOR THE HONEY-MUSTARD:

1. 1 cup mayonnaise (I used Sir Kensington's) – or use egg-free mayo for egg-free option

2. 3 tablespoons olive oil

3. 3 tablespoons raw honey (I used really raw honey)

4. 3 tablespoons Dijon mustard

5. 1 tablespoon raw apple cider vinegar

FOR THE SALAD:

1. 1 head red or green leaf lettuce, washed, patted dry and torn into bite-size pieces

2. 1 pint cherry tomatoes, cut in half lengthwise

3. 2 avocados, cut into bite-size pieces

4. 1/2 English cucumber, cut into bite-size pieces

5. 1/4 cup pumpkin seeds (soaked and dehydrated or sprouted preferred)

INSTRUCTIONS

1. Place the chicken in a large baking dish. Whisk together the lemon juice, olive oil, garli,c and sea salt and then pour over the chicken. Marinate at room temperature for 1 hour.

2. Heat grill pan over medium heat for 2 minutes. Grill the chicken until cooked through. You can also grill on an outdoor grill. Cool for 10 minutes and then cut into bite-size pieces.

3. Place the mayo, olive oil, honey, Dijon, and apple cider vinegar in a blender and blend until smooth. The dressing makes more than needed for just one salad, so store the leftovers in a Mason jar in the fridge. You can use it for other salads or as a dip for vegetables or chicken nuggets.

4. Place the lettuce, cherry, tomatoes, avocado, cucumber, pumpkin seeds, and chicken in a large salad bowl and dress with the honey-mustard dressing.

Delicious & Easy Thyroid-Friendly Apple Crisp Recipe

Ingredients

1. 6-8 Granny Smith applies, peeled & sliced

2. ¾ cup Brown sugar

3. ½ cup Flour

4. ½ cup Oats

5. ¾ tsp Cinnamon

6. ¼ tsp Nutmeg

7. 4 oz Coconut oil

8. ¾ cup Walnuts, chopped

Instructions

1. Preheat oven to 375ºF. Grease a 9 inch round Pyrex pie dish with coconut oil.

2. Place sliced and peeled apples in bottom of pie dish.

3. In a bowl, combine the brown sugar, flour, oats, cinnamon, nutmeg and coconut oil. Mix well. Add the walnuts and mix to combine. Sprinkle over the apples.

4. Bake for 30–40 minutes.

Broccoli Soup

Ingredients

1. 2 tablespoons olive oil extra virgin

2. 1 cup broccoli florets

3. 1/4 cup celery chopped

4. 1/4 cup carrots chopped

5. 2 red onions sliced

6. 1 tablespoon ginger-garlic paste

7. Salt to taste

8. 1 teaspoon of pepper

9. 1 teaspoon paprika

8. 1/2 teaspoon cumin powder

9. 1 cup of vegetable broth

10. 1/2 cup of coconut milk

11. 1 tablespoon of lemon juice

Instructions

1. Heat olive oil in a saucepan. Add sliced onion and ginger-garlic paste. Cook for 2 minutes.

2. Now add broccoli, celery, and carrots. Sprinkle salt, pepper, paprika, and cumin powder. Sauté for 5 minutes.

3. Now add vegetable broth and coconut milk. Cook on low heat for 10 minutes. Then take a hand blender and blend the soup.

4. Cook for another 3 minutes. Add lemon juice. Turn off the heat.

5. Serve.

Lemon Chicken Broccoli Sheet Pan Meal

INGREDIENTS

1. 1 ½ lbs. Broccoli florets

2. 3 tbsp. Extra virgin olive oil, divided

3. 1 tsp. fine sea salt, divided

4. Freshly ground pepper, to taste (omit for AIP)

5. 2 cloves garlic, minced, divided

6. 1 ½ lbs. boneless skinless chicken breasts

7. ½ lemon, juice only

8. Equipment needed: 1 large rimmed sheet pan, 1 large mixing bowl, 1 mini food processor or blender

Parsley Garlic Sauce:

9. 1 large bunch flat-leaf parsley, roughly chopped (about 2 cups)

10. 1 large lemon, zest and juice

11. ⅓ cup extra virgin olive oil

12. 4 cloves garlic

13. 2 tsp. Italian seasoning/herb blend

14. 1 to 1 ¼ tsp. fine sea salt

15. Freshly ground pepper, to taste (omit for AIP)

16. 1 tbsp. Water

INSTRUCTIONS

1. Preheat oven to 425 F.

2. In large mixing bowl toss the broccoli florets with 2 tablespoons olive oil, ½ teaspoon salt, freshly ground pepper (omit for AIP), and 1 clove of minced garlic. Spread evenly on large rimmed baking sheet. Place in center of preheated oven and roast for 10 minutes.

3. Meanwhile, cut the chicken breasts into 1-inch pieces, and add to large mixing bowl along with 1 tablespoon olive oil, 1 clove of minced garlic, ½ teaspoon salt, freshly ground pepper (omit for AIP), and the juice of ½ lemon. Toss to combine.

4. Remove broccoli from oven and toss with spatula. Rearrange and spread broccoli evenly on sheet pan. Nestle the chicken pieces amongst the florets. Return to sheet pan to oven for 12 to 15 minutes more, or until chicken is cooked through.

5. Meanwhile, prepare the Parsley Garlic Sauce: In a mini food processor or blender combine all sauce ingredients. Pulse to blend and mix until you reach a rustic sauce consistency. Taste and adjust with additional salt, pepper,

or lemon juice as needed.

6. When chicken and broccoli are done, remove from oven, drizzle with Green Sauce and serve.

Vitamin A for Thyroid and Sweet Potato Flour Crepe Recipe

Ingredients

1. ½ cup buckwheat flour

2. ¼ cup + 1 TBSP DHOW sweet potato flour

3. 1 TBSP coconut sugar

4. 2 TBSP ground flax seeds

5. 1 TBSP oil (I used macadamia oil) plus extra for frying

6. 2 tsp vanilla extract

7. Pinch salt

8. 2 cups almond milk (or milk of choice)

Method

1. Combine all the ingredients into a large bowl. Whisk together until well combines and a thick but runny crepe mixture forms. Allow the mixture to sit for 5 minutes

before using. This will allow the flax seeds to gel and thicken the mixture which will make it easier to flip without breaking.

2. Lightly grease a crepe pan or large frypan with oil. I use a macadamia oil spray.

3. Using a ladle spread out the batter in a thin layer coating the pan, turning the pan to spread the mixture evenly.

4. Cook on medium heat for a few minutes until the edges become golden brown, flip and cook for a few more minutes. Remove from heat and set aside.

5. Repeat until the batter is finished.

6. Serve with desired toppings, I used a vegan chocolate hazelnut spread and bananas.

Roasted Bell Pepper And Tomato Soup

INGREDIENTS

1. 1/4 cup raw cashews (soaked)

2. 1 yellow onion (chopped)

3. 4 cloves garlic

4. 4 medium vine-ripened tomatoes (stemmed, deseeded, and chopped)

5. 2 large red bell peppers (stemmed, deseeded, and chopped)

6. 1 medium carrot (peeled and roughly chopped)

7. 2 - 3 tablespoons extra virgin olive oil

8. 1 1/4 teaspoons Himalayan salt (plus more to taste)

9. 1/4 teaspoon black pepper (plus more to taste)

10. 3 - 4 cups vegetable broth

11. 3 tablespoons tomato paste

12. 1/8 teaspoon cayenne pepper (omit if Pitta)

13. 2 teaspoons nutritional yeast (omit if Pitta)

14. Roasted chickpeas (to garnish)

15. Fresh chopped cilantro or parsley (to garnish)

INSTRUCTIONS

1. Preheat the oven to 400 degrees F.

2. Toss all vegetables with the oil, salt, and pepper and spread evenly on a large rimmed sheet pan lined with parchment paper. You may need to use two sheets to avoid overcrowding of the vegetables.

3. Place in the oven and roast for 30-40 minutes.

4. Meanwhile, heat vegetable broth, tomato paste, cashews, optional cayenne, and brewers yeast in a large soup pot over medium heat.

5. Transfer roasted vegetable into the pot and simmer for 5 minutes.

6. Puree the soup using an immersion blender or carefully transfer to a blender and puree a few cups at a time, until smooth and creamy. Add more water if the soup is too thick.

7. Season with additional salt and pepper. Add a spoonful of roasted or sautéed chickpeas, sprinkle with freshly chopped parsley or cilantro and enjoy!

Thyroid-Friendly Pear & Chard Smoothie

Ingredients

1. 1 cup (250 ml) coconut water

2. ½ cucumber

3. 1 pear, cored

4. ½ lemon, peeled

5. 1 handful of chard (silverbeet)

6. 1-inch (2.5 cm) ginger

Directions

1. Wash and prepare all produce.

2. Add ingredients to blender and blend on high for 45-60 seconds until smooth.

Thyroid Health Smoothie

INGREDIENTS

1. 3 Brazil nuts

2. Small bunch of coriander

3. 1 pear chopped roughly

4. 1 orange peeled

5. 2 T pumpkin seeds or sunflower seeds

6. ¼ c yoghurt regular or coconut

7. Opt: a pinch of kelp powder

INSTRUCTIONS

1. Slice unpeeled pear crosswise, and poke out seeds with a butter knife. Peel orange or tangerine. Blend

all ingredients in your Omniblend until smooth, adding water if needed to liquify.

Red Lentil Rainbow Soup

INGREDIENTS

1. 2 tablespoons grass-fed ghee or unrefined coconut oil

2. 1 large yellow onion, chopped

3. 1 1/2 tablespoons minced garlic (about 5 cloves)

4. 2 tablespoons finely minced ginger root

5. 2 teaspoons coriander

6. 2 teaspoons cumin

7. 2 teaspoons turmeric

8. 1/8 - 1/4 teaspoon cayenne, or to taste

9. 4 cups chicken bone broth (see notes for vegan option)

10. 1 (14-ounce) can diced tomatoes

11. 1 cup dried red lentils

12. 1 medium sweet potato, peeled and diced (about 2 cups)

13. 2 1/2 ounces fresh spinach, roughly chopped (about 2 cups)

14. 1 cup coconut milk (canned, full-fat)

15. 2 scant tablespoons lemon juice

16. 1 teaspoon fine sea salt

17. 1/2 cup fresh cilantro leaves, for garnish

INSTRUCTIONS

1. In a large soup pot melt the ghee or coconut oil over medium-high heat. Add the onion and cook, stirring, until the onion is beginning to turn golden brown in spots.

2. Add garlic, ginger, and dry spices to the onion, and cook, stirring, about 2 minutes more or until very fragrant.

3. Add chicken broth, tomatoes, lentils, and sweet potato to the pot. Bring to a simmer, cover, and cook 30 minutes or until lentils and sweet potato are beginning to soften.

4. Stir in spinach, coconut milk, lemon juice, and sea salt. Taste and adjust seasoning with more lemon, cayenne, and/or salt, as desired. Turn off the heat, cover, and let sit 20 minutes more. Serve hot topped with fresh cilantro.

"Caramel" Nut Chocolate Bark

INGREDIENTS

1. 4 oz dark chocolate chopped (soy and dairy-free)

2. 1 oz. Brazil Nuts, very roughly chopped (approx. 8 med.)

* 2 oz. Medjool dates, pitted and chopped into 1/4-inch pieces (approx. 4 med.)

* 1/2 teaspoon chia seeds

* 1/4 teaspoon coarse sea salt (like Maldon)

INSTRUCTIONS

1. Melt chocolate in a double boiler, or in microwave at 30-second intervals (stirring after each), until smooth.

2. Stir in chopped Brazil nuts and dates, and spread evenly on a sheet of parchment. Sprinkle with chia seeds and sea salt, and let harden at room temperature for at least 4 hours. Cut or break into pieces and store in an airtight container for up to two weeks.

Iodine-Rich Fish Stew

Ingredients

* 1 tablespoon Butter

* 1 tablespoon olive oil

* 2 medium Yellow onions, chopped

* 1 teaspoon Coarse ground Celtic sea salt

* 1/4 teaspoon Ground black pepper

3. 1/8 teaspoon Crushed red pepper flakes

4. 1 cup White vermouth or white wine

5. 2 pounds White fish cut into chunks (I used halibut in the video)

6. 1 bunch Flat-Leaf Italian parsley, chopped

7. 1 15 ounce Can crushed tomatoes

8. 8 cups Fish bone broth, warmed homemade or store-bought

Instructions

1. Saute onions in butter and olive oil with salt and both peppers in a large soup pot. Once onions are translucent, deglaze pan with white vermouth and simmer for a few minutes.

2. Add fish and quickly saute for about 1 minute, just to cook exterior of fish.

3. Add parsley and tomatoes to pot and stir well to mix.

4. Add warm fish bone broth to pot and bring to a simmer. Simmer for 1 minute.

5. Ladle fish stew into individual serving bowls and serve with crusty baguette slices. Enjoy!

Blueberries and Lemon Cream

INGREDIENTS

1. 1 (14 oz can) organic, full-fat coconut milk

2. 1 1/2 teaspoons finely grated lemon zest (about 1 med lemon)

3. 2 tablespoons freshly squeezed lemon juice

4. 3 tablespoons maple syrup, divided

5. 1/2 teaspoon vanilla extract (for AIP sub. 1/4 teaspoon vanilla bean powder or omit)

6. Pinch fine sea salt

7. 1/2 - 2/3 cup frozen wild blueberries, thawed

8. 1 1/2 teaspoons unflavored grass-fed beef gelatin

9. 1/4 cup filtered water

10. A few mint leaves for garnish, optional

INSTRUCTIONS

1. In a blender combine coconut milk, lemon zest, lemon juice, 2 tablespoons maple syrup, vanilla (or vanilla bean powder for AIP), and salt.

2. In a small saucepan, sprinkle gelatin evenly across the surface of the water, so all granules are wet. Let the granules sit for at least 1 minute. Place over medium-low

heat and cook, stirring, just until gelatin is completely dissolved.

3. Add gelatin mixture to ingredients in blender. Blend on lowest speed, 1 minute, or until silky smooth. Pour into a medium mixing bowl, cover, and refrigerate for at least 6 hours, or overnight. This is also a good time to place your frozen berries in the fridge to thaw.

4. When ready to serve, beat the cream vigorously with a whisk until smooth and fluffy. Spoon cream into 4 (8 oz.) glasses, wine glasses, or parfait glasses. Combine thawed berries with remaining 1 tablespoon maple syrup. Drizzle berries and their juice atop the cream. Garnish if desired, and enjoy.

Pineapple Cilantro Smoothie

Ingredients

1. 3/4 cup water

2. Juice of 1 lime

3. 1 cup greens (kale or spinach)

4. 1 cup of frozen pineapple chunks

5. 1/4 of an avocado

6. 1/4 cup of cilantro

7. Small Slice ginger

8. ice

Instructions

1. Combine all ingredients and blend well.

BRAISED BEANS WITH TOMATOES AND HERBS

INGREDIENTS

1. 1 cup dried cannellini beans, soaked overnight* (you could also use white navy beans)

2. 1 cup dried chickpeas, soaked overnight

3. 2 tablespoons unsalted butter or ghee

4. 1 onion, chopped

5. 3 cloves garlic, chopped

6. 2 stalks celery, chopped

7. 24 ounce jar crushed tomatoes

8. 4 cups chicken stock

9. 3 sprigs fresh rosemary

10. 3 sprigs fresh thyme

11. 1 head Lacinato kale, chopped (you could use chard if you prefer)

12. 2 teaspoons Celtic sea salt

13. 1/2 teaspoon freshly ground black pepper

14. 1/4 cup grated Pecorino Romano cheese (optional)

INSTRUCTIONS

1. Place the cannellini beans and chickpeas in a large bowl. Cover with water and add 2 pinches of baking soda. Let soak overnight at room temperature.

2. The next day, drain and rinse the beans. Melt butter in a large pot over medium heat. Add the onion, garlic and celery and cook until just tender, about 5 minutes. Add the crushed tomatoes, chicken stock, drained and rinsed beans, rosemary and thyme and bring to a boil. Reduce the heat to a simmer and let cook until the beans are tender, about 4 hours.

3. About 20 minutes before serving, bring a pot of water to boil and add the kale to the boiling water. Cook for 8 minutes and then drain. (This step removes the goitrogens which can inhibit the uptake of iodine in the thyroid. For a

video explaining the benefits of this, check out my Instagram feed page and see my IG story titled "kale")

4. When the beans are tender, stir in the cooked kale, sea salt and black pepper. Sprinkle with Pecorino Romano and serve.

Maca Chocolate Chip Cookies

INGREDIENTS

1. 1 cup gluten free flour

2. 1/2 cup rolled oats

3. 1/4 teaspoon salt

4. 1/2 teaspoon baking powder

5. 2 teaspoons maca powder

6. 1 flax egg (see notes for instructions)

7. 1/3 cup coconut sugar

8. 1/3 cup maple syrup

9. 1/4 cup almond butter

10. 2 tablespoons olive oil

11. 1/2 cup dark chocolate chips

12. Flaky sea salt (optional)

INSTRUCTIONS

1. Preheat oven to 350°.

2. Whisk flour, oats, salt, baking powder, and maca powder.

3. In a separate bowl, make your flax egg (see notes for more information).

4. Combine the sugar, maple syrup, almond butter, and olive oil with the flax egg.

5. Combine the dry ingredients and chocolate chips with the wet ingredients.

6. Scoop cookies into balls (I used a small cookie scoop), and flatten slightly using the back of a spatula.

7. Bake for 8-10 minutes. 8 minutes for a more gooey texture.

8. Let cool. Sprinkle with flaky sea salt, and enjoy!

Apple cake

Ingredients

1. 1 cup vegetable oil

2. 4 tablespoons unsalted butter, melted

3. 2 large eggs, beaten

4. 2 cups granulated sugar

5. 2 teaspoons vanilla extract

6. 1/2 pound about 3 baking apples, such as Braeburn, Granny Smith, or McIntosh, peeled, cored, and cut into 1/4" dice

7. 1 cup chopped pecans

8. 3 cups all-purpose flour

9. 1 teaspoon kosher salt

10. 1 teaspoon baking soda

11. 1 teaspoon ground cinnamon

Instructions

1. Preheat the oven to 350°F and lightly grease a 9×13 pan or a 12-inch cast-iron skillet.

2. In a large bowl, stir by hand the oil, melted butter, eggs, sugar, and vanilla. Stir in the apple and pecans. Add the flour, salt, baking soda, and cinnamon to the bowl, and then stir until combined. Please note that this is a very thick batter, in fact it's more like a cookie batter. And while it may seem like it's unable to contain the apples, don't worry, it will be fine.

3. Spoon the batter into the baking pan or skillet, patting down the top so it's even. Bake for 40-45 minutes until the top is lightly browned and an inserted knife comes out clean.

Tuna Macaroni Salad

INGREDIENTS

1. 8 ounces Gluten-free Macaroni (like Jovial)

2. 1 cup sweet green peas, fresh or frozen (thawed), or sub. thinly-sliced sugar snap peas)

3. 3/4 cup Clean Mayo (such as Primal Kitchen or Soy-free Vegenaise)

4. 1 tablespoon dijon mustard (make sure it's gluten-free)

5. 1 1/2 teaspoons honey

6. 2 tablespoons finely minced shallot

7. 1/2 cup finely chopped fermented pickles or pickle relish (like Bubbie's)

8. 1 tablespoon lemon juice, freshly squeezed

9. Freshly ground pepper, to taste

10. Celery salt, to taste

11. 2 (4-ounce) cans low mercury tuna, (like Safe Catch Elite or Wild Planet Skipjack), or sub. canned wild salmon

INSTRUCTIONS

1. Boil pasta (8 oz.) according to package directions. With approximately 2 minutes of cooking time remaining, add peas to the boiling pasta. You may need to momentarily increase the heat to return the pot to a boil.

2. When pasta is tender, drain pasta and peas. Rinse under cold water until chilled. Drain thoroughly and set aside.

3. In a large mixing bowl, combine mayo, mustard, honey, shallot, pickles (or relish), lemon juice, pepper, and celery salt. Whisk thoroughly to combine. Taste and adjust seasoning as desired. Add tuna and mix thoroughly.

4. Add pasta and peas to tuna mixture and stir to combine. Taste, once again, and adjust seasoning as desired.

5. If possible, refrigerate for 1-2 hours before serving. Keeps 2-3 days, refrigerated.

A Thyroid-Friendly Guacamole Salad Recipe

Ingredients

For the Salad

1. 2 avocados, chopped

2. 2 Lebanese cucumber, chopped

3. 2 cups of cherry tomatoes (I used a rainbow cherry tomato mix)

4. 1 small red onion, finely chopped

5. 1 red pepper, deseeded and chopped

6. 2 scallions, chopped

7. ½ cup of japalenos (pickled)

8. 1 bunch of fresh coriander, chopped

For the Dressing

1. 2 tbsp of lime juice

2. 1 tbsp of apple cider vinegar

3. 4 tbsp of extra-virgin olive oil

4. Salt and pepper to taste

Directions

1. Wash and prepare the salad ingredients and mix into a bowl.

2. Prepare dressing — combine the ingredients together and add extra olive oil if needed. Season with salt and pepper.

3. Drizzle the dressing over the salad and mix in and enjoy!

Thyroid-Friendly Greens and Carrot Juice

Ingredients

1. 1 apple, cored

2. 1 handful green-leaf lettuce

3. 3 to 4 sprigs each cilantro and parsley

4. 4 carrots

5. ½ lime, peeled

6. 1-inch piece of ginger

Directions

1. Wash and prepare produce: Core the apple and peel the lemon.

2. Add ingredients through the juicer.

Egg Roll in a Bowl

INGREDIENTS

1. 1 1/2 pounds of pastured ground pork or grass-fed ground beef

2. 1 teaspoon fine sea salt, plus more to taste

3. White pepper, to taste

4. 1 tablespoon toasted sesame oil

5. 1/2 medium yellow onion, diced

6. 1 tablespoon freshly minced garlic

7. 1 tablespoon freshly minced ginger

8. 1 teaspoon Chinese 5-spice powder

9. 1 teaspoon ground coriander

10. 1/4 - 1/3 cup Coconut Aminos

11. 2 tablespoons rice vinegar (sub. white wine or cider vinegar for Paleo)

12. 6 cups finely chopped cabbage (about 1/2 small head)

13. 3 medium carrots, shredded on a box grater (about 2 cups)

14. 4 green onions, divided

15. Optional: 1/3 cup toasted slivered almonds for garnish

16. Optional: Serve with Sky Valley Sambal Oelek (for those who like it spicy)

INSTRUCTIONS

1. In a large, deep skillet, over medium-high heat combine the meat, 1 teaspoon salt, and pepper, to taste. Cook, stirring and breaking into small pieces, until browned, about 5 minutes. Remove from pan with a slotted spoon and set aside. Drain all but 1 tablespoon of rendered fat from the pan.

2. To the skillet, over medium heat, add the toasted sesame oil, onion, garlic, and ginger. Cook, stirring, until fragrant, 2 - 3 minutes. Add spices, coconut aminos, vinegar, cabbage, and carrots to the pan. Increase heat to medium-high and cook ,stirring occasionally, until veggies are tender, and cabbage has cooked down a bit, about 5 to 7 minutes.

3. Add browned meat back to the skillet along with half of the green onions, and stir to combine. Taste and adjust seasoning as desired with salt, white pepper, more coconut aminos and/or more vinegar. Top with remaining green onions and toasted almonds for crunch (optional), and enjoy! If desired, stir in or serve with Sambal Oelek at the table for those who like it spicy!

Homemade Granola for Thyroid Nutrition

Ingredients

1. ½ cup pumpkin seeds

2. 1 cup pecans, chopped

3. ½ cup almonds, sliced

4. 1 cup coconut, shredded

5. ¼ cup coconut oil

6. ¼ cup honey

7. 2 tsp cinnamon

8. ½ tsp nutmeg

9. ½ cup of dried apricots, chopped

How To Make

1. Preheat the oven to 350 degrees F.

2. Grease the bottom of a baking sheet with coconut oil.

3. Mix all of the ingredients, excluding dried fruit. Toss well.

4. Spread evenly on the baking sheet.

5. Bake for 15 minutes, stirring occasionally, being careful not to burn.

6. Remove from the oven and stir in dried apricots.

7. Let cool and store in an airtight container.

Hypothyroidism Smoothies Recipes

The Green Smoothie That Nourishes Your Thyroid

Tools

• Blender

Ingredients

• 2 cups coconut milk

• 1 cup chopped kale

• 1 cup fresh spinach

• 1 cup frozen chopped pineapple

• 2 T almond butter

• 1 T flax seeds

Instructions

• Combine all ingredients in a blender and pulse on high speed for 20 seconds.

• Divide between two glasses and enjoy!

Thyroid-Friendly Pear & Chard Smoothie

Ingredients

- 1 cup (250 ml) coconut water
- ½ cucumber
- 1 pear, cored
- ½ lemon, peeled
- 1 handful of chard (silverbeet)
- 1-inch (2.5 cm) ginger

Directions

- Wash and prepare all produce.
- Add ingredients to blender and blend on high for 45-60 seconds until smooth.

Transformational Green Smoothies for Hashimoto's

Ingredients

- A handful of spinach or mixed greens
- 1 cup full-fat coconut milk
- 1/4 green apple chopped

• 1/2 cucumber peeled & chopped

• 1/4 cup frozen wild blueberries dark cherries, or raspberries

• 1/2 avocado peeled

• 1 scoop pea protein non-denatured whey protein, or Hydrobeef protein

• 1 scoop PaleoFiber or TruFiber

• Ice cubes if desired, for a creamy consistency

• Optional: Maca powder turmeric powder, collagen powder, MSM powder, cacao powder, Camu Camu powder, carnitine tartrate, PaleoGreens, PaleoReds, Chia seeds, ground flaxseed, flax oil, and/or inositol powder

Instructions

• Add liquid to the blender and add protein powder, fruits/veggies, additional fiber, optional ingredients and blend. Add ice cubes if desired, and blend a few more seconds.

• Enjoy.

Chocolate Protein Smoothie

INGREDIENTS

• 1 frozen Banana (Ripe is recommended for sweetness)

• ½ cup light coconut milk

• ½ cup coconut water

• 1/2 cup ice cubes

• 1 tablespoon almond butter

• 1 tablespoon cacao powder

• 1 to 2 scoops of your favorite protein powder*

• A pinch of fine sea salt

• 1 tablespoon chia or flaxseed (optional)

INSTRUCTIONS

1. Place all ingredients except chia or flaxseed in blender. Blend on high until smooth.

2. Optional: After blending stir in 1 tablespoon chia or flaxseed and let sit 10 minutes (so seeds can gel) before enjoying.

Thyroid-Friendly Greens and Carrot Juice

Prep Time: 5 minutes

Total Time: 5 minutes

Servings: 1

Serving Size: 16 to 20 ounces

Ingredients

- 1 apple, cored

- 1 handful green-leaf lettuce

- 3 to 4 sprigs each cilantro and parsley

- 4 carrots

- ½ lime, peeled

- 1-inch piece of ginger

Directions

- Wash and prepare produce: Core the apple and peel the lemon.

- Add ingredients through the juicer.

Energy Boosting Tropical Turmeric Smoothie

Prep Time: 1 minute

Cook Time: 4 minutes

Total Time: 5 minutes

Servings: 2

Ingredients

- 2 cups organic chard or spinach optional
- 2 cups organic coconut, almond or hemp milk
- 2 cups fresh or frozen organic pineapple
- 1 cup fresh or frozen organic mango
- Juice of ½ organic lemon
- ½ to 1 tbsp fresh, grated organic ginger to taste
- 1 tsp ground organic, non-irradiated turmeric
- ¼ tsp fresh ground black pepper

Instructions

- Throw all the ingredients in a blender and voila!
- Use at least one frozen fruit to make smoothie cold.

Notes

1. Adding the chard or spinach makes this smoothie a real powerhouse but note, it will turn the smoothie green.

Banana And Peanut Butter Smoothie

INGREDIENTS

- Banana - 1 overripe and frozen overnight
- Peanut butter - 1 tbsp
- Milk of choice - 1 cup 200ml
- Steel cut/rolled oats - 1 tbsp
- Sweetner of choice - optional
- Ice cubes - 4-5 nos

INSTRUCTIONS

- Blend all the ingredients into a mixer and pour into a glass.
- Serve chilled.

Banana Orange Creamsicle Protein Smoothie

INGREDIENTS

• 3 navel oranges, peeled and thickly sliced, seeds removed

• 3 bananas, frozen

• 14 oz can light coconut milk (or your preferred DF milk)

• Collagen peptides and/or your preferred protein powder

• Optional: chia seeds, or ground flax (omit for AIP)

INSTRUCTIONS

1. In a blender combine oranges, frozen bananas, coconut milk and collagen hydrolysate. Blend on high speed until smooth and frothy.

2. Optional: Stir in chia seeds or ground flax. Enjoy.

Thyroid-Friendly Mediterranean Juice

Prep Time: 5 minutes

Total Time: 5 minutes

Servings: 1, 16 ounce (500 ml)

Ingredients

- 1 red pepper, seeded

- 1 tomato

- 1 lemon, peeled (optional)

- 1 cucumber

- 4 sprigs oregano

- Pinch sea salt (optional)

Directions

- Wash all produce well

- Cut off stem of red pepper and remove seeds

- Peel lemon if desired, or if the lemon isn't organic

- Slice cucumber and tomato to fit your juicer

- Juice all ingredients, wrapping oregano around cucumber to get best yield. Juice stems with oregano for maximum flavor.

- Garnish with oregano leaves, lemon slice and pinch of Himalayan or sea salt.

Almond Banana Cinnamon Smoothie

Prep Time: 2 minutes

Cook Time: 3 minutes

Total Time: 5 minutes

Equipment

• Blender

Ingredients

• 4 bananas

• 4 cups almond milk

• 2 tbsp vanilla extract

• 1 cup almond butter

• 1 tbsp cinnamon

• 10-15 ice cubes

Instructions

• Combine all ingredients in blender except ice. Run for a couple seconds till everything is blended.

• Start adding the ice cubes a couple at a time. Blend until smooth.

• Add more ice cubes if you like a thicker smoothie.

Horchata Chia Pudding

INGREDIENTS

• 1 (14-ounce) can light coconut milk

• 1/2 teaspoon almond extract

• 1/2 heaping teaspoon cinnamon

• 1/3 cup chia seeds

• 1/4 teaspoon stevia powder (or sub. 2 tbsp. maple syrup)

• Optional Toppings: Fresh berries, toasted sliced almonds, toasted coconut

INSTRUCTIONS

1. Shake the can of coconut milk well before opening and pouring into a medium mixing bowl.

2. Add remaining ingredients and whisk vigorously to combine, until no lumps remain.

3. Taste and adjust sweetness as desired. Cover and refrigerate for at least 4 hours or overnight.

4. Serve with your toppings of choice. Keeps refrigerated for up to 5 days.

How to make a smoothie – the basics

Equipment

• Blender

Ingredients

• 1 scoop of plant protein powder OR 2 tbsp of a combination of high protein seeds like hemp or chia seeds

• 1/2 cup total mixed fruit frozen makes the smoothies so much creamier and more delicious, but you can use fresh

• ¾-1 cup of liquid depending in the thickness you prefer of choice (usually chilled almond milk, coconut milk, coconut kefir, or organic yogurt or goat's milk if you eat dairy)

• 1-2 tbsp of a healthy fat often a nut butter which adds protein, too

• Optional your nutrient boosts

Instructions

• Blend all ingredients in a blender until smooth.

Hormone Balancing Smoothies

Ingredients

Chunky Monkey Smoothie

- 1.5 cups dairy-free milk

- 1/2 large banana

- 1 tbsp cashew butter

- 1 serving (scoop) unflavored collagen peptides

- 1 tbsp cacao powder

- 2 tsp maca powder (optional)

- 2 tsp cinnamon (optional)

- 2 tbsp chia seeds or acacia fiber

- 2 handfuls spinach leaves (about 2 cups)

Creamy Berry

- 1 1/4 cup dairy-free milk

- 1/4 cup berries (any mixture of blueberries, raspberries, strawberries, etc.)

- 2 tbsp chia seeds

- 1 serving vanilla protein powder

- 2 tbsp walnuts

- 2/3 cup frozen cauliflower rice

- 2 handfuls spinach leaves

Lean and Green

- 1 1/4 cup dairy-free milk

- 1/3 cup diced zucchini

- 1/4 large avocado

- 1/4 cup diced kiwi

- 3 tbsp hemp seeds

- 1 serving vanilla protein powder

- 2 handfuls chopped kale leaves

Instructions

• Place ingredients for whichever smoothie you choose into your blender. Do this in the order they are listed in the ingredients section. Blend until smooth (you may need to pause halfway and scrape down the sides), this could take 2-3 minutes. If smoothie is too thick to your liking, add in additional milk by 1/4 cup.

Healthy Strawberry Smoothie with Yogurt

PREP TIME: 5 minutes

COOK TIME: 0 minutes

TOTAL TIME: 5 minutes

SERVINGS: 1 smoothie

CALORIES: 107 kcal

EQUIPMENT

• Blender

INGREDIENTS

• 1 cup strawberries frozen or fresh

• ½ cup nonfat Greek yogurt

• Handful ice

• Stevia to taste

INSTRUCTIONS

• Add all ingredients to a blender.

• Blend until smooth then transfer to a glass and enjoy

NOTES

• If using fresh strawberries, add more ice to smooth it out more.

• This is a thick smoothie, you can add more ice to thin it out.

• If you want to add more protein, add a scoop of protein powder with 20 to 30 grams of protein and thin with more ice or milk.

Apple Cucumber Smoothie with Protein and Variations

PREP TIME: 5 minutes

COOK TIME: 0 minutes

COURSE: Breakfast, Drinks, Snack

SERVINGS: 1 CALORIES

Calories: 383 kcal

EQUIPMENT

• 1 cutting board

• 1 chef knife

• measuring cups and spoons

• 1 blender

INGREDIENTS

• 1 cup milk higher in protein such as cow's, soy, or pea milk

- 1 apple

- 1 small cucumber or ½ of a large cucumber

- ½ avocado

- ½ cup plain Greek yogurt

- ½ cup ice

- 1 tablespoon maple syrup or honey, or 1 to 2 pitted and chopped dates

INSTRUCTIONS

- Core and chop the apple and place it in the blender.

- Roughly chop the cucumber and place it in the blender.

- Add the remaining ingredients to the blender as well as any optional ingredients you'd like to add and blend until smooth.

Blueberry Detox Smoothie

Prep Time: 15 minutes

Servings: 1 Smoothie

Calories: 693kcal

Equipment

• Vitamix High-Speed Blender

Ingredients

• ½ cup frozen wild blueberries

• ¼ cup frozen cranberries

• ¼ lemon with rind rind is optional but recommended

• 1 tablespoon almond butter or seed butter see post

• 1 tablespoon pumpkin seeds

• 1 tablespoon chia seeds

• 1 tablespoon hemp seeds

• 2 walnuts

• 2 Brazil nuts

• ¼ avocado peeled

• ½ tablespoon coconut butter see note

• ½ cup unsweetened almond milk or hemp milk

• ½ cup water optional, or extra almond milk

Instructions

• Soak the pumpkin seeds, chia seeds, hemp seeds, walnuts, and brazil nuts in the almond milk for at least 30 minutes. This will activate the enzymes for easier digestion. I usually do this step when I first wake in the morning.

• Combine all the ingredients in a high-speed blender and blend on high speed until smooth.

• You can leave it thicker, pour into a bowl and eat with a spoon as shown.

• Or, add enough water, or additional almond milk, so that the smoothie is drinkable to your taste.

Berry Smoothie

INGREDIENTS

• 1 cup frozen strawberries

• 1 cup almond milk

• Handful of ice cubes 4 or 5

• 1 apple

• Handful of frozen blueberries

• 1 1/2 cups Greek yogurt

• Unsweetened flaked coconut to garnish

INSTRUCTIONS

• In a high speed blender, blend all ingredients together until smooth. Add ice to the blender and blend or you can serve over ice in a glass. Enjoy immediately.

High Protein Chocolate Banana Smoothie

INGREDIENTS

• 1 cup almond milk

• 1 banana about 1/2 cup frozen

• 2 tbsp raw cacao powder

• 3 tbsp collagen hydrolysate gelatin or raw organic hemp protein for vegan

• 1 tbsp almond butter or tahini

• 1 tsp coconut oil

• 1/2 tsp maca optional- this is great for balancing hormones

• 1/2 tsp apple cider vinegar optional

• 1 tsp vitamineral green optional- this is a great way to include some extra vitamins and minerals

INSTRUCTIONS

• Place all ingredients in a high powered blender. I prefer the vitamix because it's so powerful and can be used for almost everything. The blendtec is also a good option.

• Blend on high until all ingredients are blended. Add ice or water to desired consistency

Keto Smoothie Recipe with Avocado, Chia Seeds & Cacao

INGREDIENTS

• 1–1¼ cups full-fat coconut milk

• ½ frozen avocado

• 1 tablespoon nut butter of choice

• 1 tablespoon chia seeds, soaked in 3 tablespoons of water for 10 minutes

• 2 teaspoons cacao nibs, cacao powder or cocoa powder OR 1 scoop of chocolate protein powder made from bone broth

• 1 tablespoon coconut oil

• ice (optional)

• for topping: cacao nibs and cinnamon

• ¼ cup water, if needed

INSTRUCTIONS

1. Add contents into a high-powered blender, blending until well-combined.

2. Top with cacao nibs and cinnamon.

Strawberry Protein Shake

- Prep Time: 5 minutes
- Total Time: 5 minutes
- Category: Breakfast
- Diet: Gluten Free

INGREDIENTS

- 1 cup raw milk or (1/2 cup coconut milk and 1/2 cup water)
- 1 cup frozen strawberries
- 1/4 teaspoon raw honey (optional)
- 1 teaspoon vanilla extract
- 1 scoops Mama Natural Collagen Peptides
- 2 raw egg yolks (optional)
- A few slivers of raw, frozen liver (optional – see post above about why I use this ingredient)

INSTRUCTIONS

1. Place all ingredients in a blender and blend until smooth.

Cucumber Lime Veggie Smoothie Recipe

PREP TIME: 5 minutes

TOTAL TIME: 5 minutes

CALORIES: 222kcal

Servings: 2 smoothies

Ingredients

• 2 cups water (or coconut or almond milk for a more creamy smoothie)

• 1 cucumber (roughly chopped)

• 2 cups fresh spinach

• 2 limes (juiced)

• 2 kiwi (peeled and chopped)

• 1 tsp fresh ginger (peeled and chopped)

• 1 tsp matcha powder optional

• ½ fresh avocado (skin removed)

• ½ cup frozen pineapple or fresh plus some ice cubes

• 1 scoop greens powder (optional, but adds a lot of extra nutrients)

• 1 scoop collagen powder (optional)

Instructions

• Place water or milk, cucumber, and spinach in a blender and blend until completely smooth.

• Add remaining ingredients and blend on high again until completely smooth.

• Serve immediately and enjoy.

Healthy Apple Pie Smoothie

Ingredients

• 1 red apple cored, peeled and chopped

• 1 frozen ripe banana peeled prior to freezing, sliced

• ¼ cup rolled oats or quick oats

• 2 Medjool dates pitted

• ⅓ cup almond milk or favorite plant-based milk

• 1 tablespoon maple syrup

• ½ teaspoon vanilla extract

• ½ teaspoon ground cinnamon

• ⅛ teaspoon ground ginger

• ⅛ teaspoon ground nutmeg

Instructions

• Add all ingredients to a blender.

• Blend all the ingredients until the chunks of fruit are gone and the smoothie is smooth and creamy.

• Taste and adjust to taste. Add some additional maple syrup if you want it sweeter.

• Transfer the smoothie to a cup, top with cinnamon and serve.

Gingerbread Smoothie Recipe

INGREDIENTS

• 1 banana

• 1/2 cup coconut milk or almond milk

• 1/4 avocado

• 2-3 tbsp collagen protein or hemp protein for vegan

• 1 tbsp coconut oil

• 1 1/2 tbsp molasses

• 1/2 tsp cinnamon

• 1/4 tsp ginger powder

• 1/8 tsp cloves

• 1/2 cup baby spinach optional- for added nutrients!

• ice to desired consistency

INSTRUCTIONS

• Place all ingredients into a high powered blender then blend. Add water or more dairy free milk if needed. Once the smoothie is blended into a puree, add ice to reach desired consistency and blend.

30-Day Nutritional Meal Plan for Hypothyroidism

Day 1: Monday

1. Breakfast: Start with a spinach and berry smoothie blended with Greek yogurt and chia seeds.

2. Lunch: Enjoy a quinoa salad topped with grilled chicken, avocado slices, and a refreshing lemon vinaigrette.

3. Dinner: Indulge in baked salmon accompanied by roasted sweet potatoes and steamed broccoli.

Day 2: Tuesday

1. Breakfast: Begin the day with oatmeal topped with sliced bananas, walnuts, and a drizzle of honey.

2. Lunch: Relish a turkey and avocado wrap in a whole-grain tortilla, served with a side of crunchy carrot sticks.

3. Dinner: Warm up with a hearty lentil and vegetable soup paired with whole-grain bread.

Day 3: Wednesday

1. Breakfast: Delight in a Greek yogurt parfait layered with fresh berries, almonds, and a sprinkle of cinnamon.

2. Lunch: Enjoy a chickpea salad mixed with spinach, cherry tomatoes, cucumber, and feta cheese, dressed in a tangy balsamic vinaigrette.

3. Dinner: Savor grilled chicken breast alongside quinoa pilaf and roasted Brussels sprouts.

Day 4: Thursday

1. Breakfast: Energize with scrambled eggs cooked with spinach and tomatoes, served with whole-grain toast.

2. Lunch: Treat yourself to a tuna salad featuring mixed greens, quinoa, chickpeas, and a zesty lemon-tahini dressing.

3. Dinner: Dive into stir-fried shrimp with a medley of vegetables and nutty brown rice.

Day 5: Friday

1. Breakfast: Indulge in a vibrant smoothie bowl topped with granola, sliced kiwi, and shredded coconut.

2. Lunch: Enjoy a refreshing Caprese salad composed of mozzarella cheese, tomatoes, fresh basil, and a drizzle of balsamic glaze.

3. Dinner: Delight in baked cod with quinoa salad and sautéed kale.

Day 6: Saturday

1. Breakfast: Start the weekend with whole-grain pancakes topped with Greek yogurt and a medley of mixed berries.

2. Lunch: Wrap up grilled vegetables and hummus in a whole-grain tortilla, served with a side of crisp mixed greens.

3. Dinner: Enjoy turkey meatballs in marinara sauce served over zucchini noodles.

Day 7: Sunday

1. Breakfast: Begin the day with overnight chia seed pudding made with almond milk, topped with sliced strawberries and coconut flakes.

2. Lunch: Relish spinach and quinoa-stuffed bell peppers paired with a fresh side salad.

3. Dinner: Conclude the week with a savory beef stir-fry featuring broccoli, bell peppers, and nutty brown rice.

CONCLUSION

The hypothyroidism diet stands as a vital strategy in managing the complexities of thyroid dysfunction. By focusing on nutrient-rich foods that are high in iodine, selenium, zinc, and essential vitamins, this dietary approach aims to optimize thyroid function and overall health. It places emphasis on achieving a balanced intake of macronutrients, reducing inflammation, and promoting gut health, all of which are crucial in effectively managing the symptoms associated with hypothyroidism.

Beyond its nutritional benefits, the hypothyroidism diet promotes sustainable lifestyle changes that support long-term health. By incorporating a variety of wholesome foods such as lean proteins, vegetables, fruits, whole grains, and healthy fats, individuals can stabilize energy levels, manage weight effectively, and potentially mitigate the risk of complications linked to untreated hypothyroidism.

Choosing to adopt the hypothyroidism diet, with guidance from healthcare professionals, empowers individuals to take charge of their well-being. It offers a proactive approach to enhancing thyroid function, improving overall quality of life, and fostering lasting habits that contribute to vitality and health resilience. Integrating this dietary regimen into a comprehensive treatment plan provides practical strategies for managing thyroid health and underscores the importance of nutrition in achieving and maintaining optimal well-being.

9 798332 683411